THE INTERSECTION BETWEEN PAIN AND PURPOSE

BY

WILLIE J. LIGHTFOOT SR.

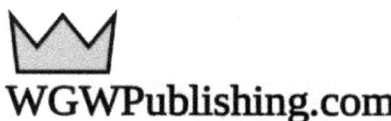

WGWPublishing.com

Copyright © Willie J. Lightfoot Sr. 2023

All Rights Reserved

ISBN: 979-8-9852535-9-7

Cover Art: Damian Brown, Afficial Inc.

Editing: Wandah Gibbs, Ed. D.

Printed in the USA

WGW Publishing, Inc. Rochester, NY

FOREWORD

Willie J. Lightfoot Sr. was born destined for public service. The son and namesake of a dedicated and determined community activist, he has seen up close from early childhood, a model of positive public service. He also learned first-hand that progress is hard won, and not without difficulty and challenge. It was no secret to him that opposition and resistance can sometimes overwhelm progress. Based on these types of situations, Mr. Lightfoot skillfully learned to strategize and articulate a plan for overcoming such challenges, and developing plans for how to move forward in a positive and strategic way.

The paths he has chosen for his career trajectory have been instructive, as well as inspirational; a military veteran of foreign conflicts, a public servant and first-responder, an elected official who has served multiple terms without the hint of scandal or corruption, a successful entrepreneur and community developer who continuously gives back to his community, and a pastor and denominational leader.

In many of his pursuits, Willie Lightfoot experienced pain and disappointment, all the while keeping focused on the things that give his life spiritual purpose. He is a person of great integrity and an inspiration to young and old alike. In writing *The Intersection Between Pain and Purpose,* he is to be commended for translating the life lessons he's learned over the years into a plan for successful living. It is a plan of action as much as it is an aspiration and inspiration.

Just one of his titles and positions would command full-time attention, though he has held several of them simultaneously. Through it all, he has been a devoted husband and father who always puts the interests of his family first. He is a loving husband to Verdina Lightfoot. They have been together for 30 years and married for 26 of them. They have four adult children, three grandchildren, and an English Bulldog named Sapphire.

---William A. Johnson, Jr.
64th Mayor of Rochester NY (1994-2005)

I dedicate this book to my entire family; my wonderful wife of 30 years, my children, grandchildren, my mother, my sister, my brother, all my aunts, uncles, and my cousin.

I wish to honor both my late father, the Honorable Willie Walker Lightfoot and my late stepfather John Thompson.
Rest in power Kings!

I also want to mention my dearly, (albeit tragically), departed dog Pearl. Our wonderful 10-year-old Chinese Shar-Pei, was viciously murdered by two Pitbulls who broke through our fence, then attacked and killed our family dog in her own backyard. This horrific event was an extremely traumatic event for our entire family.

INTRODUCTION

As a pastor, councilman, business owner, and community activist, I was moved to write this book after recognizing the level of pain, trauma and dysfunction that exist in my cherished community. Pain and trauma can paralyze people, preventing them from thriving and reaching their full potential.

Inspired by my own experiences and trauma, I wrote this book in the hopes of reaching people where they are in their healing process. My goal is to empower people to acknowledge their pain and to understand that ultimately, there is a godly purpose to their suffering. The Bible teaches us in the book of Romans, Chapter 8:28, "All things work together for good to them that love the Lord, and who are called according to His purpose."

I've come to recognize that much of the pain I've endured and the trauma I've witnessed, have ultimately catapulted me towards my destiny and purpose. Also, along the way, I noticed that everyone can identify with loss. Each of us has lost someone or something. Lost job opportunities, lost health, lost family members, lost innocence, lost friends, lost joy, and peace.

One of the greatest traumas I experienced was that of losing my late father, the Honorable Willie Walker Lightfoot. This man, who was larger than life and who paved the way for me in this world, left a huge void when he passed. Many people never recover or find it very difficult to recover from the loss of a loved one and the associated trauma. I can attest to the intense pain to those times when it feels like we'll never experience joy again. I'm here to tell you however, that God is ever present and that He is patient and close to the broken-hearted. I can also tell you the grief cannot be rushed, avoided nor side-stepped. Grief is a journey that must be travelled. There comes a time along that road however, that by the grace of God, we realize the pain we've been experiencing is not as intense as it once was and that the void our loved one left is slowly filling up with joyful memories as we reminisce about them. God is able to restore your joy and He will one day use you to comfort someone else as they mourn the loss of a loved one.

The Coronavirus pandemic of 2020 and the post pandemic trauma have been extremely challenging. Many have lost loved ones, have suffered the pain of isolation and have had to deal with loneliness and fear. I pray this book encourages us to evaluate pain and loss from a different perspective and helps us understand that pain can in fact intersect with our purpose. May we recognize opportunities to bring healing to those who are still hurting and be a resource for individuals suffering in silence through trauma and pain. We are extremely resilient and able to walk through grief to a place of joy and healing. God is patient and kind and He has given us the tools to endure and to experience the joy of healing. Beginning today, and using the tools God provides us, let's begin to consider and explore our pain and trauma in a new light. Let us embrace our journey and experiences and begin to view them as opportunities to understand where our pain intersects with our purpose…

TABLE OF CONTENTS

THE PAIN	2
THE SCARS	34
THE HEALING	76
THE PURPOSE	92
THE PRAISE	114
ABOUT THE AUTHOR	136
RESOURCES	142

PART 1

THE PAIN

THE PAIN

Many of us have done a very good job of masking our pain. We've practiced it, we've lived it, and we've buried it because the pain is so intense. Revisiting it takes us to a deep dark place so we prefer to ignore it.

We're getting ready to dive into this pain thing and as we do, we may unlock some sealed chambers. There are many layers to this topic that many of us can identify with. Layers are often compounded on top of each other. As we peel back those layers you may find yourself strongly identifying with feelings you've never faced before. If that occurs that's great, and though this is the beginning of your healing journey, you may find you need to see your pastor or a counselor to help you navigate through to the other side.

As people of color, our healing is often delayed or out of reach as we've made it taboo to receive counseling. Certainly, rooted in our complicated and difficult history, there are reasons counseling has been ignored as a valuable path to wholeness, however counseling and therapy are valuable tools for each and every one of us.

The Bible tells us not to stand in the counsel of the ungodly, therefore we can assume that the opposite would be to stand in the council of the godly. It's absolutely okay to seek help. As we go through this five-part series and peel away layers, we don't want to leave people's wounds exposed and vulnerable.

Everybody needs somebody to talk to, somebody you can call at 2 or 3 o'clock in the morning. Someone who'll take the time and who is not going to say, "I told you so," nor beat you over the head with advice. We all need somebody who'll just listen. When it comes to pain, sometimes we just need to talk about it and get it out. We just want somebody to listen and say, "I love you and I'm here for you." At times like these we need an encourager instead of someone who's going to condemn us or judge us or put our business in the streets.

Beloved, do not be surprised at the fiery trials when it comes upon you to test you as though something strange were happening to you, but rejoice and so far as you share Christ's sufferings that you may also rejoice and be glad when His glory is revealed. If you are insulted for the name of Christ, the spirit of glory and of God rests upon you, but let none of you suffer as a murderer or as a thief or as an evildoer. If any one of you suffers as a Christian, let him not be ashamed but let him Glorify God in that name. For it is time for judgment to begin in the household of God and if it begins with us, what will the outcome be for those who do not obey the gospel of God and if the righteous is scarcely saved, what will become of the ungodly and the sinner? (1 Peter, Chapter 4).

Chronic pain is defined as long-lasting pain. Some people have been in pain for a very long time. They've suffered pain over and over again, both neurological and/or physical pain. Perhaps the pain is the result of a physical injury or some sort of medical disorder. However, not all pain is physical but rather emotional or psychological. Some may suffer with mental health disorders or deal with family members who suffer with mental health disorders.

The loss of a loved one can be extremely painful. The hurt associated with losing a loved one can run so deep that some never fully recover. I remember when my father passed away over 20 years ago. The pain was extremely intense and though my wife is my best friend, my father was my first best friend. He was my hero, my mentor and someone I could always rely on. He was always there; whether I needed to borrow $20, needed a ride across town or even a place to stay.

Though I know we're not supposed to put our faith in man, losing a parent, a brother or sister, a spouse or a child is devastating. There's tremendous emotional pain that comes with such loss which can take us to really dark places. Feelings of; anger, despair, sadness, suicide, fatigue, depression, and anxiety are not uncommon while grieving.

Grieving is a necessary part of the healing process, and must take its course. However, sometimes the pain is so intense that we need help in finding a strategy through to the other side. Pain and sadness after loss are completely normal, but feeling like we no longer want to go on or getting stuck in our sadness is not healthy or productive.

Pain is defined as something we feel physically, emotionally or psychologically. Bottom line, when we think of pain, each of us can say we've experienced it on some level. I've certainly experienced it in my life in one form or another. I've felt it both physically and emotionally.

It should be noted however, that pain is not the same for everyone. The intensity may be higher or lower for some and pain may be temporary or chronic. Some pain is buried and manifested in different ways. We may not have had the same types of painful experiences, but each of us can acknowledge that we've been hurt in some way or another. If you've never experienced hurt, I would submit to you that if you keep on living you will eventually experience some hurt and pain.

The bible tells us that we're going to suffer as Christians. We're going to suffer persecution. We're going to suffer pain. You're going to have some, "Why am I going through this pain?" I got saved. I'm not supposed to be going through pain anymore right?. Well, the bible tells us that you're definitely going to go through pain. Just because you're a child of God does not mean you're exempt from pain. What it does mean is that God will comfort you, never leave you nor forsake you and He will see you through.

Question is: How do we show up every day? Ask yourself: How do I show up every day? We either use our pain for our purpose or we allow it to overtake us.

II Corinthians 4:8-18

"We are troubled on every side yet not distressed. We are perplexed but not in despair, persecuted but not forsaken, cast down but not destroyed, always bearing about in the body the dying of the Lord Jesus Christ that the life also of Jesus Christ might be made manifest in our bodies."

We must understand that we're going to be persecuted. We're going to be treated a certain way just because of what we believe, who we believe in and because of what we stand for. "But greater is the one that is in you than the one that is in the world!" (1 John 4:4).

I want you to know saints of God and friends that because you have God in you, the devil can't stand you. The enemy will come at you in many forms and pain is just one of them. The devil will try to abort your purpose by causing your pain to get in the way of your purpose instead of fueling it. The very reason the enemy comes at you is because he wants to discourage you. The reason the enemy is trying to hurt you is because he wants to prevent you from reaching your purpose.

Other times, your greatest enemy, your greatest foe are those of your own household. Sometimes, the greatest source of pain are those that love us the most or those who are supposed to love us the most and who are supposed to be our protectors and our providers. There's no worse pain than that which is caused by church folks and family.

Many people especially women, have been mistreated. Bad relationships, divorce, verbal and emotional abuse. You don't always have to be hit upside your head in order for it to hurt. Some people have been hit upside their head with words. Words hurt deeply and leave bruises and scars. They say, "Sticks and stones will break your bones but words will never hurt you." Well guess what, we now know that that's not true. Words can hurt you. Words have power and can traumatize you. Imagine being told you'll never amount to anything or that you're stupid or ugly, or can't do anything right. After a while you start to believe it.

Many of us grew up going to church. We went to Sunday school, went to vacation bible school, and were in the choir. We were around church people all the time. Most are good God-fearing folks and are wonderful friends, prayer warriors and people who walk in joy and humility. We are taught that church is where we should be and where we can feel safe, but I would be remiss if I did not point out that we now know that a tremendous amount of pain and abuse has occurred in churches. Because it is so unexpected, it really messes people up.

God has revealed to me that there are a lot of people who have experienced church related pain. Some have been molested in the church. People have been mistreated in the church. Others have been robbed in the church. A number of them have been cussed out. People have been looked down on or overlooked in church. People may have been mistreated, not only by other churchgoers, but also by deacons, preachers, Sunday school teachers, and choir directors. Some church leaders have behaved unseemly and abused their position in the church. They've hurt people which is extremely confusing because these are the very people the saints look up to.

Often, the very one who's been abused loved God with great zeal and had purpose. Then, their innocence was challenged when somebody said something foul or mistreated them. One bad situation or occurrence in church has run off many a church member and prevented them from walking in their purpose. I get it, but the horrible acts of one person are not enough to separate you from the love of God nor can it permanently prevent you from walking in your purpose. I'm here to tell you that what happened to you was wrong and must be acknowledged and dealt with, but your resulting pain will still somehow serve a purpose.

You are not alone and the isolation and shame one feels after such events can be crippling where your spiritual walk is concerned. Obviously I can't speak specifically about your situation or family, but I can speak of my own. I have family members who were molested when they were children. Back in the day, we did not necessarily have the words or the tools to deal with such abuse and unfortunately they are still carrying the pain. They are now in their

60's and 70's and are still hurting and still showing up with that same unresolved pain.

I ask you today, saints and friends, how are you? Are you showing up carrying pain? Are you showing up carrying unforgiveness? Have you admitted to the fact that pain is affecting your quality of life?

We tend to bury pain but It's not something you can permanently cover up or mask. It will eventually manifest in other ways. Pain is not something that just goes away. Some of us have "locked" the pain away in our spirit and in our mind because addressing it, causes too much trauma. We don't even want to think back to that time in our life because it's too difficult.

Now I know what you're thinking, "Preacher, the bible tells us to forget those things which are behind and press towards the mark of the high calling in Christ Jesus," but the fact of the matter is; if you're showing up mean, mad and ugly, and lashing out at other people, then you haven't "forgotten those things which are behind…" If you carry around a spirit of ugliness, a spirit of hate and a spirit of meanness, there's something inside of you, that you have not yet been delivered from! Ouch!!! There's something inside of you that hasn't been set free and that is keeping you enslaved to anger and pain.

Remember, your pain has purpose. God can turn it around. Men are evil but God is good. Men have free will and there are times when some do horrible things. But whatever happened to you when you were a child, God is able to bring healing and help you regain your joy, your strength and to feel His love again. God will show you that he can heal your scars and massage your wounds. God knows and understands your pain. He's able to take you through the hurt and bring you out.

God has healed many of you. He has restored your joy, has brought about forgiveness, has given you a new walk and a spring in your step. Some of the most beautiful Christians have been through so much, yet were able to work through their pain to receive God's grace and healing. You'd be surprised at some of the testimonies people have. If we knew what they went through, we'd be all the more amazed at God's healing power. Those who've truly dealt with their pain now embody this scripture: "The joy of the Lord is my strength."

Pain is like luggage, it becomes heavy and more burdensome the longer you carry it around, particularly because we end up carrying it with us everywhere we go. If you've got pain in your heart that you've not dealt with, you're actually carrying it with you to church, to work, to the mall, into restaurants. Hurt people hurt other people. It shows up in the way you talk to people, how you treat people. Sometimes the pain shows up before you do! And whenever you open your mouth, out comes PAIN!

Have you ever met mean Christians? They're saved, sanctified and supposedly filled with the Holy Ghost. The Bible tells us we're supposed to have a spirit of meekness, that we're supposed to be humble, slow to speak, and swift to hear. We're not supposed to be walking around in the spirit of anger or jealousy, instead we're to be treating people with love.

So, when you scratch your head and wonder, "Lord, these people here in church say they're saved, sanctified and filled with the precious Holy Ghost, then why are they showing up looking and sounding like the devil?"

How can you preach without a smile? How can you sing without joy? How can you teach without the spirit of love? How can you carry yourself in such a way that you're not even trying to act like Jesus? He was meek, He was lowly, yet He was the King of Kings and the Lord of Lords. He has all power to destroy the earth and the power to do anything He wants, yet He walked in his purpose, fulfilling the will of the Father.

Pain plays a significant role in our purpose and our pain helps shape us into who we are. Our pain makes us or breaks us. We must first acknowledge that it exists and then we have to deal with it. Don't sweep it under the rug, don't ignore it or act like it isn't there or that the cause of the pain never happened. Deal with it. I know this is tough, but you've got to come from amongst the hidden places of pain and out into the open.

To do so, some of you will need to reach out for counseling, and that's okay. We want to draw you out of that place that caused you so much pain and that is causing your quality of life to suffer. I want you to realize that pain plays a significant role in your health, in your relationships, friendships, and even at work. We've got to acknowledge the hurt and we've got to deal with it. Don't let anyone tell you: "Just get over it." You must first acknowledge that you've been hurt, that you've got this pain, and that your heart has been broken.

The Bible tells us to come boldly before the throne of grace. When we come to God, it's okay to come clean. After all, he already knows all about it. He just wants you to acknowledge it so He can heal you and deliver you in such a manner that you realize that all of your help comes from Him. All we have to do is say something along these lines, "God, you know, my heart has been broken, but I'm here to acknowledge it and to admit that I need healing. I need your help Lord, and I need your healing touch upon my heart. I ask Lord that you heal my pain and that you allow it to intersect with my purpose."

Identifying pain and how it intersects with our purpose, helps us to lean intentionally into it, which then helps us to understand our purpose.

SRIPTURE REFERENCES & RECAP

1 Peter 4:12-19

"Beloved, do not be surprised at the fiery trial when it comes upon you to test you, as though something strange were happening to you. But rejoice insofar as you share Christ's sufferings, that you may also rejoice and be glad when His glory is revealed. If you are insulted for the name of Christ, you are blessed, because the Spirit of glory and of God rests upon you. But let none of you suffer as a murderer or a thief or an evildoer or as a meddler. Yet if anyone suffers as a Christian, let him not be ashamed, but let him glorify God in that name. For it is time for judgment to begin at the household of God; and if it begins with us, what will be the outcome for those who do not obey the gospel of God? And If the righteous is scarcely saved, what will become of the ungodly and the sinner?"

Job 30:17

"The night racks my bones, and the pain that gnaws me takes no rest."

Revelation 21:4

"He will wipe away every tear from their eyes, and death shall be no more, neither shall there be mourning, nor crying, nor pain anymore, for the former things have passed away."

WHAT IS PAIN?

Merriam Webster Definition: **(1):** a localized or generalized unpleasant bodily sensation or complex of sensations that causes mild to severe physical discomfort and emotional distress and typically results from bodily disorder (such as injury or disease).

THE FIVE COMMON TYPES OF PAIN::

1. Acute pain
2. Chronic pain
3. Neuropathic pain
4. Nociceptive pain
5. Radicular pain

These describe physical pain but I would submit that in the long run, all pain ends up affecting us physically. Therefore pain, though it presents as physical, may have resulted from some other form of pain such as physical or emotional.

This leads us into our next point which describes some of the side effects of pain.

MENTAL HEALTH DISORDERS!
(YES, MENTAL HEALTH IS A REAL THING)

- Anxiety disorder
- Attention deficit disorder
- Bipolarity
- Borderline personality disorder
- Depression
- Eating disorder
- Generalized anxiety
- Obsessive-compulsive disorder
- Panic disorder
- Post-traumatic stress disorder
- Schizophrenia
- Social phobia

THE EFFECTS OF PAIN

How do we show up every day? How do I show up every day? We've all dealt with some type of pain and we've either used it for our purpose or it has overtaken us.

2 Corinthians 4:8-18 (KJV)

"We are troubled on every side, yet not distressed; we are perplexed, but not in despair; Persecuted, but not forsaken; cast down, but not destroyed; Always bearing about in the body the dying of the Lord Jesus, that the life also of Jesus might be made manifest in our body."

THE ROLE OF PAIN

Pain plays a significant role in our purpose. Our pain shapes us into who we are. Our pain is what makes us or breaks us. We have to acknowledge our hurt and our pain and we must deal with it and not sweep it under the rug. We must address the elephant in the room, the hurt.

Let's begin by asking ourselves:

How is my pain affecting my quality of life? Lord help me to acknowledge that this pain exists, then help me to deal with it.

Jesus is the prime example of how pain intersects with purpose:

Isaiah 53: 4-6

"Surely he took up our pain and bore our suffering, yet we considered him punished by God, stricken by Him, and afflicted. But He was pierced for our transgressions, He was crushed for our iniquities; the punishment that brought us peace was on Him, and by His wounds we are healed. We all, like sheep, have gone astray, each of us has turned to our own way; and the Lord has laid on Him the iniquity of us all."

I Peter 2: 21-23

"To this you were called,-because Christ suffered for you,-leaving you an example, that you should follow in His steps. He committed no sin, and no deceit was found in His mouth. When they hurled their insults at Him, He did not retaliate; when He suffered, He made no threats. Instead, He entrusted himself to Him who judges justly."

COUNSELING AND THERAPY

Sometimes, to help us sort out our pain, we need to talk to someone who specializes in that sort of thing. This person can help us identify the pain, the source, and the effects it is having on our lives. Though God is our ultimate healer and counselor, a well-trained counselor or therapist can show us the pathway towards healing.

Types of Counselors:

- Marriage and family counseling
- Guidance and career counseling
- Rehabilitation counseling
- Mental health counseling
- Substance abuse counseling
- Educational Counseling

NOTES

Have you suffered pain in your life? How did it make you feel?

_____
_____
_____
_____
_____
_____
_____
_____
_____
_____
_____
_____
_____
_____
_____
_____
_____
_____
_____
_____

List any other thoughts you had while reading this Chapter:

_____
_____
_____
_____
_____
_____
_____
_____
_____
_____
_____
_____
_____
_____
_____
_____
_____
_____
_____
_____
_____
_____
_____

PART 2

THE SCARS

SCARS

Our purpose in this lesson is to realize why it is important to acknowledge that we have scars. Though scars are a topic that may be difficult to talk about, it is fundamental to do so along the journey towards healing and forgiveness. Whether our scars be physical or whether they be spiritual; either way, we want to continue to lean into our pain, acknowledge our scars, heal, and learn how they might intersect with our purpose.

Scars are reminders and indicators of pain. Even Jesus Christ did not come to new life without scars, the wounds, and the marks of his struggle with darkness. Instead of being wiped away by divine power, those scars became the evidence of His risen life. The wounds left by His suffering and His death on the cross become the identifying marks of God's goodness and love.

The same goes for us. At times, we wrestle with the dark times of our lives. After our struggles with darkness, scars remain as identifying marks of the God who takes our weaknesses and transforms them into strengths. He takes our failures and turns them into victories. After all, Jesus had scars on His hands and He had scars in His side as reminders of His great sacrifice, His suffering and His purpose.

We must learn to be real with ourselves. It helps to recognize that each of us has some form of emotional and/or spiritual scarring. It's something we can all identify with and trust me, if you didn't have many scars before, it's safe to say that following the Coronavirus Pandemic lockdown and isolation, we all have some. The Covid-19 pandemic had an impact on each of our lives and we've all been scarred emotionally on some level...

For starters, and for a long time during the lockdown, we couldn't even come to church. We couldn't hold church services like we used to or gather together like we needed to. We had to walk around with masks on and even had to be careful while gathering with our own family members. Some of us could no longer visit our elderly friends and relatives and sadly, many of them died in forced isolation. This caused extraordinary pain and trauma in families all over the world. Though the Swine Flu of 2009 was declared a pandemic by the World Health Organization, we'd never experienced a pandemic of the Covid-19 magnitude in this century. It was frightening and for many, traumatizing.

Most of us know that the Bible says, "Forsake not the assembling of yourselves with the saints." We know the word tells us to assemble ourselves with our brothers and our sisters. The Bible also tells us that when two or three touch and agree, our prayers will be answered. There's something very important about touching a person's hand during prayer or hugging someone upon greeting them.

Ironically, during this very emotional, challenging and stressful time, we probably needed physical contact and emotional reinforcement more than ever, but were required to isolate and keep our distance instead. For most of us, we couldn't leave the house at all during the mandatory lockdown for fear of catching and or spreading Covid-19.

First, we need to understand what scars are. Emotional scars sometimes go unseen, but over time, when people haven't dealt with the cause of their scarring, signs begin to appear on their face, especially in their eyes.

While mandated to wear protective masks in public during the pandemic, the only thing we could see was each other's eyes. Remember, the eyes are the windows to the soul and often times, when we look into a person's eyes, we are able to detect scars.

You can actually see pain. You can identify anguish and sometimes you can detect unforgiveness. You can actually recognize the strain and results of scarring and how it has taxed their self-esteem. Usually, scars involve some kind of rejection or put down especially when coming from those we love and trust. Has anybody ever been let down in life? Has anybody ever been rejected? Have any of you ever been hurt by somebody you loved and somebody you trusted? Others may have grown up in a home filled with negative criticism? When disapproval becomes part of everyday life, it's emotionally damaging and usually leaves significant scars.

Maybe you grew up in a home where you were told you were too fat; you were not needed or that you were cross-eyed. Maybe you were body-shamed and told you didn't look like a certain somebody else in the family or you didn't walk like somebody else or talk like somebody else. I'm talking about somebody that grew up in a situation where you were constantly picked on, or constantly bullied.

You were hurt emotionally and let me tell you; people say, "Sticks and stones may break my bones but names will never hurt me," but I want you to know that name-calling does hurt. It sure does and if we are to be honest with ourselves, derogatory insults hurt deeply. They cut deep down in the bowels of our soul, especially when they come from someone we love.

I believe that the entire church family will be in a better place when we can identify our hurts and admit they occurred. "You know what? You're right, I've been hurt. Hurt emotionally, hurt psychologically, mentally, and spiritually."

The remaining scars are generally a result of attacks on our self-esteem. Many people are walking around with low self-esteem especially following this pandemic. We're seeing more homelessness than ever before amongst our youth and amongst older people. I'm seeing faces I've never seen before out in the streets. The shelters and missions are full. People are hurting. People's self-esteem has hit an all-time low, often times because of the isolation and rejection they've endured.

The church is supposed to be a place of acceptance. The church is supposed to be a place where you bring people in, a place of positive injection, not rejection. We're supposed to be injecting the spirit of Jesus Christ into all we come in contact with. Oh, but let me tell you, for someone who grew up surrounded by negative criticism, it takes a long time to work through the destruction that criticism caused.

Why is it that in the later years of life some of us are still tormented by things that were said to us as children? Perhaps you were talked to by a loved one or a parent or maybe even by a preacher or someone that you esteemed highly. Maybe it was someone you cared about deeply, but to this day you still remember the pain associated with something they said to you.

Though it takes a long time to work through this type of destruction, it is possible. By being open to healing and remaining committed throughout the process, every individual can become that person God wants him or her to be. And though the scars caused by put downs and criticism may remain, in time with God's love, kindness and patience, you can definitely find healing and work through most of it.

Jesus went to the cross, was crucified, then resurrected, but as you see in the scriptures, His scars remained. Spiritual scars arise when God's blessings are obscured from us. This often happens because some significant person in our lives expressed doubt or disapproval or killed our creative dreams. We start to believe that no one believes in us.

Have your dreams been shattered? You had a dream to start a business, to play football. You had a dream and the devil sent somebody to squash it. Don't you know, that in the same way God works through people, the devil can too?

That's why we must be careful of what we say to people. Beware of the dream-snatcher. Don't snatch somebody else's dream. Think about it: because of doubt or disapproval during our lifetime, we sometimes attribute the same attitude unto God. We believe that God disapproves of us in the same way others have. Maybe He did not want us to do this or that, or He's displeased with this outcome or that outcome. Or perhaps our parents raised us to be afraid of God so we kept our distance from divine affairs.

Jesus appeared to His followers after His resurrection with a peaceful, comforting demeanor, thus addressing their immediate need for reassurance. Jesus even invited Thomas, also known as *Doubting Thomas*, to touch His scars. The disciples rejoiced when they recognized Jesus because of his scars. This encouraged and empowered them to move on with their lives. New life comes out of pain and scars.

Scars are not easy to deal with but must be acknowledged so a wound can heal. A scar needs to be tended to and exposed to light and air. Physical scars are easier to expose whereas emotional and spiritual ones are more difficult to deal with because of the shame associated with them. What will people think of me once they find out I have a drinking problem? Or a drug problem? What will they think of me once they know I have a gambling disorder? When they discover I have a sexual addiction, or indulge in sexual immorality? What will they think of me when they know I have unresolved problems? Will they ridicule me? Will they resent me? Will they use me for a punching bag and beat up on me or judge me? What will people do when they find out about my scars? Well guess what: we ALL have scars of one sort or another that we've towed around for years.

Also, let it be known that there is a difference between a scar and a scab. A scab appears at the beginning stages of healing. Have you ever had a scab you kept picking at? You kept picking at it and messing with it and before you know, it started to bleed again and wouldn't heal properly or as quickly as it should. Many of us have been in such a position where we're picking at a wound or allowing other people to pick at it and therefore it's not healing as it should.

On the other hand, some of us are not healing properly because we keep getting reinjured. We keep getting hurt again and again; returning to the same place of pain, the same place we incurred the scars in the first place.

During the healing process, know that you might have a scab that itches and might even be painful for a while, but it is part of the journey towards wholeness.

This might apply to someone on drugs or someone trying to give up alcohol. Or it could be you in an abusive relationship. But Jesus can heal your wounds, your scabs and lead you to a safe place.

Three things to consider:

- ➤ Scars are signs and indicators of past injury and pain
- ➤ There is a difference between scabs and scars
- ➤ Along our journey towards healing, we may encounter what we call *triggers*.

Jesus appeared after the resurrection indicating that new life comes out of our pain and scars. Nevertheless, it's not easy to deal with scars and as previously mentioned, there's a certain amount of shame associated with them. But our scars become the testimony which helps us solidify our purpose. When Thomas realizes that Jesus is indeed alive, he confesses that his Lord God is stronger and more powerful than any other. This often happens when a doubter becomes a staunch believer. Let's face it, we all have doubts and questions. Do not be afraid of these but rather seek answers and develop an intelligent, informed faith.

Our scars become identifying marks of our strengths. I think about the late actor Michael K. Williams, who starred in *The Wire* and in *Game of Thrones*. He was a well-respected artist who was tragically found dead in his hotel room in 2021. I watched a *YouTube* video he recorded years ago where he was talking about how he got that significant scar on his face. He explained that he'd gotten it during a bar fight when someone slashed him with a razor blade. Now you know, a razor blade can cut you wide open and leave a horrible scar.

He went on to explain in the video that he's not normally inclined to fight but that he'd gotten into a bar fight because he'd been drinking too much. He confessed that he'd actually caused the fight because he'd been talking junk to others in the bar. During the fight someone cut Michael's face with a knife all the way from his eyebrow to his chin.

After that incident, not only was he ashamed, but he thought his acting career might be over and he sunk into a deep depression. After some physical and emotional healing, he eventually realized that his scar actually intersected with his purpose. Because of that scar, he ended up playing a tough guy and getting cast in some really high-profile movies and TV shows.

I'm in no way advocating getting into bar fights and getting cut up, but in his case, after some healing, Michael's scar intersected with his purpose in a big way. It didn't hinder him, but instead propelled him towards his destiny. Some of you have scars that may be propelling you towards your destiny. Women can certainly relate to this when scars remain on your body because of pregnancy and childbirth. When you look at those scars, you are reminded of the wonderful blessing that came out of your body. Your scars are a living witness that you were able to carry a child and bring it into the world. A child was born and you have scars as a reminder of what you went through for nine months while carrying your baby.

Others may have a different set of scars because maybe when you gave birth, your child didn't make it. In that case, your scars take you to a totally different place. Some of you have bullet wounds. Nevertheless, over time and with healing, our scars become a reminder of how God saw us through.

Do you know that you can actually die from a BB gun pellet? Yes, it can travel through your body and cause a blood clot which can kill you. Some of you have been shot with real bullets. Perhaps it happened at age 22 or 38, or later on in your 40's or 50's and now you've got a scar. You've got a testimony of what God can do during the healing process. Some of you have scars you incurred in a car accident and now have a scar that triggers you whenever you look at it.

There's one more thing to consider when it comes to scars, scabs and triggers. What role if any, have you played in terms of scars? Are you the victim, the perpetrator or the witness? Proverbs 18:21 reads: "Death and life are in the power of the tongue and they that love it shall eat the fruit thereof."

I must confess, I was one of those kids on the bus that got a kick out of teasing and pulling on a girl's pigtails. You know, constantly clowning around. I never realized how annoying I was until later in life, after running into people I went to elementary and high school with. I've actually had to apologize to some of them because of what they told me. "Hey, remember that time on the bus?" or "You remember that time you did this or that?" Generally, I don't remember their names nor remember who they are. After all, It's been well over 30 years since I teased people in school. Clearly however, some of my victims remember me harassing them! Understand this; things we do can have a lasting impact on people's lives. We've got to be careful about what we do and say to people.

In one instance, a guy come up to me and said: "Remember when you kicked my lunch box over?" I'm thinking to myself: It's been 37 years and this is still bothering you? But you know what? I realized in that moment that I needed to be present for that person. I had to come out of my self and understand that I owed him an apology. I've apologized for stuff I did over 30 years ago. Some of you are going to have to go back and apologize for stuff you did 30 or 40 years ago because you may be the cause of somebody else's wound. That's right. Knowingly or unknowingly, you may be the one picking at their scab.

The church has to be careful also. One reason some people have church pain is because often times they go seeking help with severe trauma and the church is really not qualified to help in that capacity. Just because you're a minister doesn't mean you have a counseling degree nor does becoming a bishop mean you're a medical doctor.

When someone comes to you with a troubling issue, it's not always time to play counselor. Understand that people may have been in such a traumatic situation that something you say could trigger them instead of helping them heal. When you realize their issue is deeper and more serious than you can handle, it's important not to judge. Instead, it's a good time to refer them to the Pastor or another senior leader. Meanwhile, offer to pray for them, to stand by them and to check in on them. If you've had a similar situation or experience, acknowledge that and share your testimony of healing.

TRIGGERS

Back to the issue of triggers: I Corinthians 10:13 indicates, "There have been no temptation taken you but such as is common unto man. But God is faithful who will not suffer you to be tempted above what you can bear, but will with the temptation also make a way of escape that you may be able to bear it."

Triggers are stimuli set off by memory or trauma or a specific portion of a traumatic experience. Imagine you were trapped in a car after an accident. Then several years later, you're unable to unlock the restroom stall you're in. You might feel a surge of panic which is probably reminiscent of the accident.

Though some triggers are easily identified and anticipated, there are many that are buried, subtle and inconspicuous, often surprising an individual and catching him or her off guard. We've all been caught out there by our triggers at one time or another. It is important for us to identify potential triggers, and draw a connection between strong emotional reactions and the triggers. Then it becomes easier to develop coping strategies so we can manage those moments.

A trigger is a sensory reminder of a traumatic event, usually set off by a noise, a smell, a temperature, physical sensation, or visual scene. Triggers can generalize to any categorization no matter how remote the resemblance. Revisiting a location can trigger someone. Some people won't return to certain places because it triggers them.

Then there are some people we no longer want to be around because their language triggers us. Over time, we notice and are able to identify what our triggers are.

This is perhaps simpler for a drug addict or somebody in alcohol recovery because their obvious triggers are stress, drugs and/or alcohol. It becomes immediately clear that there are certain places and people they can no longer be around as it could trigger them into a relapse. There are even certain things they should no longer see or do.

Bear in mind that once an addict gets clean, there are probably underlying issues that need to be resolved. Perhaps someone started drinking to alleviate stress or to forget past pain. Maybe drug use began as a social thing but became something quite different. Maybe behaviors exhibited during the period of addiction are causing guilt and remorse. All that needs to be addressed in order to be free from the past. God is so able to help during this time and will send you someone you can talk to. Someone who can guide you through to the other side of your addiction.

In as much as it is relatively easy to identify addiction triggers, it is often much more difficult to identify emotional ones. Previous trauma of any sort can be triggered at any time by simply revisiting the location where the traumatic event occurred. For some, having children reach the same age at which you experienced abuse or seeing the same breed of dog that bit you or perhaps hearing loud, angry exchanges between people can set you off.

Some are triggered by a specific time of day, a season, a holiday, an anniversary, or an event. Those of you who've been through marital problems may carry your pain into the next relationship. Perhaps certain things your new partner does resembles behaviors in a previous relationship which then triggers you. There are certain signs that get your antenna up because you've seen it before. You've been down this road before. I've seen this and I know what comes next, whether true or not.

What's happening here? What's going on? Essentially, those scars, and the wounds you thought were healed, begin to swell up again. Even if your new partner hasn't done anything wrong, all these questions start swirling around in your head. What are you doing? Why are you doing it? It's because you've been triggered. There's a pain inside you that's hurting from a previous wound. There's an emotional scar unexpectedly rearing its head. On the other hand, we should be aware that sometimes something we say could trigger someone else, which could lead to violence.

FLASHBACKS

A *flashback* differs from a trigger in that it occurs when we experience previous trauma as if it were actually happening in the present. It can set off a reaction that resembles the same reaction we had during the trauma itself. A flashback experience is usually very brief and typically only lasts a few seconds but the emotional after-effects can linger for hours.

Flashbacks can be initiated by a trigger but not always. Sometimes, they occur out of the blue. Other times, a physical state increases a person's vulnerability to re-experience trauma fatigue. High stress level flashbacks can feel like a brief movie scene. Hearing a car backfire on a hot sunny day, may be enough to cause a veteran to react as if they were back on the battlefield.

Our visual nightmares and intrusive thoughts can be traumatic in and of themselves. Frequent intrusive nightmares and dreams can be exhausting and a fear of falling asleep could develop because of previous trauma which can also take a toll.

SCRIPTURE REFERENCES & RECAP

John 20:19-25 (KJV)

"Then the same day at evening, being the first day of the week, when the doors were shut where the disciples were assembled for fear of the Jews, came Jesus and stood in the midst, and saith unto them, Peace be unto you. And when he had so said, he shewed unto them his hands and his side. Then were the disciples glad, when they saw the LORD. Then said Jesus to them again, Peace be unto you: as my Father hath sent me, even so send I you. And when he had said this, he breathed on them, and saith unto them, Receive ye the Holy Ghost: Whosoever sins ye remit, they are remitted unto them; and whosoever sins ye retain, they are retained. But Thomas, one of the twelve, called Didymus, was not with them when Jesus came. The other disciples therefore said unto him, We have seen the LORD. But he said unto them, Except I shall see in His hands the print of the nails, and put my finger into the print of the nails, and thrust my hand into His side, I will not believe."

We should be aware of the difference between scars and scabs. Scars can remain permanently, whereas a scab is an indication that a wound is beginning to heal.

We also carry emotional and spiritual scars. Emotional scars are sometimes unseen, but often when people have not dealt with the causes of their scars, you can see the evidence of scars on their faces, especially in their eyes. Scars such as these are generally the result of attacks on our self-esteem. Usually, it involves some kind of rejection or put down, especially from those we love and trust.

A person who grew up in a home where negative criticism was part of everyday life is most likely emotionally damaged and scarred. It takes a long time to work through this type of destructive criticism. However, with openness and persistence, a person can become the individual that God has destined him or her to be. However, even after a person works through emotional put downs, some scars remain.

On the other hand, spiritual scars arise when we block God's blessing from our lives.

This often happens because some significant person in our life expressed doubt or disapproval of our own creative dreams and then we end up projecting that same attitude onto God. We imagine God disapproves of us too.

For example, if we have a parent whose love was conditional or made us feel that we had to do everything perfectly in order for them to show love, we may attribute that same behavior to God. If I sin or fall short of God's expectations for me, I may believe that God will withdraw His love from me. But God has unconditional love for us and the bible tells us that "He will never leave us nor forsake us." In other words, there's nothing we can do to cause Him to withdraw his unconditional love for us. God is love and he absolutely loves us no matter what. He may not like some of the things we do, but he definitely loves us.

Maybe our parents raised us to be afraid of God so we kept our distance from divine affairs. That too is a lie. We learn in I John 4:18 that "Perfect love drives out fear," and Psalm

56:3 indicates, "when I am afraid, I will trust in you Lord."

Jesus appeared to His followers after His resurrection, ministering to their immediate need for reassurance that it was indeed Him. Jesus invited Thomas to touch his scars. The disciples rejoiced when they recognized Jesus because of His scars. This encouraged and empowered them to move on with their lives.

New life comes out of the pain of our scars. Scars are not easy to deal with and before a wound can heal, it must be exposed to light and air. Physical scars are easy to expose. Emotional and spiritual scars are more difficult to deal with because of the shame generally associated with them.

OUR SCARS ARE OUR TESTIMONY AND HELP SOLIDIFY OUR PURPOSE

When Thomas believes that Jesus is alive, his confession, "My Lord and my God," is stronger than any of the others. It often happens that a doubter becomes one of the staunchest of believers. We all have doubts and questions. Do not be afraid of them. Develop an intelligent faith; a faith rooted in study and facts. Jesus offers us the same invitation he offered to Thomas. "Do not doubt, but believe!" Remember, over time and with healing, our scars become identifying marks of our strength.

Some Things to Consider:

Proverbs 18:21 (KJV)

"Death and life are in the power of the tongue: And they that love it shall eat the fruit thereof."

1. We must consider our actions as well. Was there a situation where you were

the victim? Are there times when you've been the perpetrator or the witness? What role do you play?

1 Corinthians 10:13

"There hath no temptation taken you but such as is common to man: but God *is* faithful, who will not suffer you to be tempted above that ye are able; but will with the temptation also make a way to escape, that ye may be able to bear *it*."

In some instances, to understand the purpose of your pain you must identify what role you played along the journey.

A trigger is a stimulus that sets off the memory of a trauma or a specific portion of a traumatic experience. It's important for us to identify potential triggers and draw connections between strong emotional reactions and triggers. Then we can begin to develop coping strategies to manage those moments when a trigger occurs.

A trigger is any sensory reminder of a traumatic event: a noise, a smell, temperature, other physical sensation, or visual scene. Triggers can generalize to any characteristic, no matter how remote, that resemble or represent a previous trauma, such as revisiting the location where the trauma occurred. Triggers are often associated with the time of day, season, holiday, or anniversary of the event.

A flashback is re-experiencing a previous traumatic experience as if it were actually happening in that moment. It includes reactions that often resemble the person's reactions during the trauma.

Flashback experiences are very brief and typically last only a few seconds, but the emotional after-effects linger for hours or longer. Flashbacks are commonly initiated by a trigger, but not necessarily. Sometimes, they occur out of the blue. Other times, specific physical states increase a person's vulnerability to re-living a trauma, (e.g., fatigue or high stress levels). Flashbacks can feel like a brief movie scene that intrudes on a person's thoughts.

We all have scars, and those scars have stories. Thankfully, God made the human body extremely resilient. For example, when you get a cut, your body immediately goes to work to heal it. It just happens without you even having to think about it. And often, once the body has finished its work and the wound has closed, there remains a scar where the wound was. The scar simply becomes evidence of healing.

However, when we experience an emotional wound, our body does not naturally go into recovery mode. We have to take an active role in processing what happened and asking the Lord for healing.

When we give it to the Lord, He begins to work in our heart. He eases the pain and grants us the ability to forgive the one who hurt us. An emotional wound cannot heal without forgiveness. Unforgiveness and bitterness are like an infection. You must forgive others and you must learn to forgive yourself. Once the Lord has helped you work through your pain, your life will be a compelling testimony to the power of the Holy Spirit.

OUR SCARS KEEP US FROM REPEATING MISTAKES

They help us to not repeat mistakes. They also remind us to be careful not to injure others.

Like many people, I have scars from past relationships. And while I've processed them and moved on, I dare not forget them. I don't want to repeat past mistakes in a new relationship. I don't want to ignore red flags and be injured again.

Remembering old wounds also makes me more sensitive to how I treat others. I don't let my past define me or dictate my future, but I do allow it to inform it.

My scars act like bumpers at the bowling alley. When I start heading toward the gutter (start to repeat my past mistakes), I feel the bumper (remember how I was hurt in the past) and bounce back onto the right path. Scars can keep us on track if we remember them in a healthy way.

1 Corinthians 16:13-14

"Be on your guard; stand firm in the faith; be courageous; be strong. Do everything in love."

Pray for healing of scars and wounds both past and present. Pray for understanding of our triggers and to take more notice of how we might be impacting others.

NOTES

List some of the scars you recognize in yourself. What triggers them?

_____
_____
_____
_____
_____
_____
_____
_____
_____
_____
_____
_____
_____

List any other thoughts that arose while reading this chapter:

PART 3

THE HEALING

THE HEALING

STEPS TOWARDS HEALING

First, we must acknowledge and admit that we have pain. As previously mentioned, we also want to come to grips with the fact that we most likely have scars. I've got some on my body and also have some spiritual scars in my heart and on my mind. In Psalm 51:10-12 God said, He would create in me a clean heart and would renew a right spirit within me.

The devil wants to place triggers in your path but I'm here to tell you what Philippians 2:5-11 says, "Let this mind be in you which is also in Christ Jesus," indicating that we don't have to walk after the flesh but rather walk after the spirit because it's the Spirit that's going to heal our scars. It's the Holy Spirit that's going to maneuver our way of escape despite the triggers. It's the Spirit that's going to give us what to say to a hurting person.

We all have scars and stories, and we've got to be careful how we speak to people. For example, you haven't seen someone in a long time. They've lost weight perhaps and when they walk into church, the first thing you say to them is, "You look like you done got sick." You have no idea how much they had to go through just to drop the weight they had. You don't know how many nights they sat up crying concerned about their weight. Ever stop to consider what people deal with? I'm using this example but you can apply it to a lot of situations.

You don't know how hard someone had to struggle on any given day, just to get to the church. They may have tried on five outfits simply to find something to wear which didn't make them look too overweight. Coming into the house of the Lord should feel like a place of safety, a place of refuge. It should not be a place where you'll be further traumatized or hurt.

God said he'd never leave me, never hurt me, and never abandon, yet on some days, as soon as I walk into the church, the devil tries to pull my trigger. Satan loves to point out how men and women of God act or don't act. Do you know how many people have left the church because of a trigger caused by the very people who call themselves saints. The devil loves that!

The Bible tells us in James 1:19; Everyone should, "be swift to hear and slow to speak." Proverbs 18:21 indicates; "Death and life are in the power of the tongue."

Are you an encourager? Are you a Christian? Are you a child of God? Are you the one trying to help somebody? Just remember, when you're in pain and navigating scars you haven't dealt with, it's hard for you to help somebody else. We all have scars and those scars have stories.

It must be reiterated that one cannot heal from an emotional wound without forgiveness. Unforgiveness, and bitterness are like infections that prevent a wound from healing. You must learn to forgive others and also to forgive yourself. The good news is: once the Lord has helped you work through your pain, your life becomes a compelling testimony.

Be courageous. Learn to communicate with one another. Gently tell your husband or wife what they're doing that makes you feel the way you do. If they keep hurting you and you never tell them that it hurts then they will never know. In relationships, you've got to have those difficult conversations. Tell him, "Honey, it hurts me when you say that or when you speak to me in that way."

When somebody comes up to you in church and says something offensive, you've got to be courageous and say, "You know what? You are a brother, so in all love, I need to let you know that what you just said to me, hurt me. I'd appreciate it if you didn't talk to me that way." Right then and there, you're dealing with the situation before it causes a scar. You're allowing yourself to be healed and move on.

On the other hand, if someone keeps coming at you and you never say anything and if they constantly insult you and pick at you, you'll have to remove yourself from the abuse. Emotional abuse can be spiritual abuse at first, but it's a form of bullying and abuse nonetheless.

I Corinthians 16:13 reads, "Be on your guard, stand firm in the faith, be courageous, be strong and do everything in love."

We must identify our scars and triggers, then examine ourselves and ask God to teach us, to heal us and allow us to become whole. As we navigate the healing journey, it allows us to evolve into a better person, partner and friend.

SCRIPTURE REFERENCES & RECAP

Isaiah 53:5 (KJV)

"But He was wounded for our transgressions, He was bruised for our iniquities: the chastisement of our peace was upon Him; and with His stripes we are healed."

Types of Healing:

- Physical healing (of the body)
- Emotional healing (of the heart)
- Mental healing (of the mind)
- Spiritual healing (of the spirt or soul)
- Holistic healing (of the body, heart, mind and spirit)

Jesus heals His children because He has compassion on the sick and hurting. One such occurrence is recorded in Matthew 14:13–14

"When Jesus heard what had happened, He withdrew by boat privately to a solitary place. Hearing of this, the crowds followed Him on foot from the towns. When Jesus landed and saw a large crowd, He had compassion on them and healed their sick."

Compassion moved Jesus to heal a man with leprosy (Mark 1:41–42), a boy possessed by an impure spirit (Mark 9:22), and two men who were blind (Matthew 20:34). He even raised a widow's son from the dead (Luke 7:11–17).

The feeding of the 4,000 is motivated not by a desire on Jesus' part to demonstrate that He is the bread of life, but by His compassion for the multitude (Matthew 15:32). Even the healing of the most severely demon-possessed person described in the New Testament is ultimately attributed to God's mercy (Mark 5:19).

Steps to Emotional & Spiritual Healing:

- ➤ Admission & Grieving
- ➤ Confrontation & Disclosure
- ➤ Forgiveness & Reconciliation
- ➤ Restoration & Healing

The power to receive and have complete healing lies in God.

Philippians 4:19 (KJV)

"But my God shall supply all your needs according to His riches in glory by Christ Jesus."

He provides us with the necessary resources to be healed; people, places and things.

It should be noted that there is the matter of our own healing and then there's the healing of our surroundings, community and world.

2 Chronicles 7:14 (KJV)

"If my people, which are called by my name, shall humble themselves, and pray, and seek my face, and turn from their wicked ways; then will I hear from heaven, and will forgive their sin, and will heal their land."

Healing is a journey which requires acknowledgement, sometimes it requires confrontation, forgiveness, and ultimately reconciliation. At times that requires a conversation with someone who offended you, at other times it's much more difficult to achieve.

Some conversations are more difficult than others and sometimes the offender is not willing to acknowledge they played a role in your hurt and pain. Having a 3rd party mediator present may ease the difficulty and help guide each party through a reconciliation process. A pastor, a trusted friend or unbiased family member, a counselor or therapist can be great resources.

There are other times when the one who hurt you is no longer walking this earth. Or other times, the offender is too violent, frightening or is a stranger and should definitely not be confronted. This is where God's forgiveness towards others is yours through the Holy Spirit. You may not be able to do so on your own, but with God, He will give you the power and the grace to forgive.

After all, God's grace is sufficient for us…He forgave us our trespasses and loves us unconditionally. What a wonderful gift! It stands however that forgiveness is often a process whereby we forgive someone over and over, each time the offensive memory surfaces we turn it over to God and we claim His forgiveness towards the offender.

It is not easy and can be a bit frustrating, but it is a fact that unforgiveness brings about a root of bitterness that can destroy us. Ironically, the one we need to forgive is often no worse for wear and goes about life unbothered. We on the other hand, develop anger, pain, bitterness, and an unforgiving spirit, which does us no good whatsoever. We're the only one it hurts…

Remember, God is the ultimate healer, forgiver, restorer, and way-maker. Ask Him for help forgiving an offender, a destructive family member, an abusive parent or an ex. God will show you the way to true healing, forgiveness and freedom from anger and hatred.

You got this…begin a new day by admitting and acknowledging your scars. When possible and if safe, confront and disclose to your offender. Begin the process of forgiving and, when possible or beneficial, reconciliation. That will ultimately lead to a place of restoration and healing.

NOTES

What steps are you taking to ensure you are on a journey towards your healing?

_____
_____
_____
_____
_____
_____
_____
_____
_____
_____
_____
_____
_____
_____
_____
_____

PART 4

THE PURPOSE

THE PURPOSE

Humans naturally seek answers to the following questions:

1. Who am I?
2. Why am I here?
3. Where am I going?

Ironically, besides our Heavenly Father, the one that knows us best, is the devil. He knows exactly when you became a child of God. He then tried everything he could to pull you back into darkness. I bet temptation was never a huge problem until you got saved, then all of a sudden, prospects started coming out of the woodwork. All sorts of vices, cravings, attractions, urges, and the like are amplified as Satan tries to distract us from our new nature. If that's not enough, he loves to bring up past shortcomings, addictions, mistakes, and sins.

Don't worry though, for the bible tells us that "Greater is He (God) that is in you, than he (Satan) that is in the world." (1 John 4:4) The sooner you realize that Satan is weak compared to God's spirit, love, power, and forgiveness, the sooner he will no longer be able to torment you.

When it comes to God's love and forgiveness, I'm here to tell you that it doesn't matter who you were, it no longer matters what you used to do, and it doesn't matter what sins you committed. You are now a child of God and therefore what really matters is who you are today. So, when you ask yourself; "Who am I?" The answer is: "I am a child of God," Once we realize this, we no longer walk through life trying to figure out, "Who am I?"

Of course, the enemy wants to confuse you because that's his job. He created a system rooted in confusion. But if you were to ask me who I am, I'm going to say without reservation that, "I'm a child of God." It doesn't matter what type of situation I used to be in or the type of person I used to be or the sorts of things I used to do. Once I met God, once I called upon the name of Jesus, something happened and I am a changed man. I was given a new start. God made me brand new; I have a changed mind, I have joy, I am no longer enslaved to certain vices and activities, and I am living and loving my new life in Christ.

When you gave your life to Christ, something became new in you too. People can talk about me if they want to and say, "He seems like he's acting brand new." Yeah, you're right baby, I sure am and I'm excited about it. I'm acting brand new because the Bible tells me that when I came into Christ, I became a new creation.

Before I met Jesus, I really didn't know who I was. I was moving in all the wrong directions and chasing all the wrong things. I had a mind to do wrong, but I thank God that He created a clean heart in me and He renewed my spirit.

Some of you used to be on drugs, used to run the streets, and were whoremongers. Some of us used to be liars, deceitful, and manipulative. Others were full of pride, rude, unforgiving, full of jealousy and envy. You see, all sin is sin and all of us are born with the original sinful nature. But that's precisely why Jesus died and rose again, thus providing the pathway to salvation and setting us free from our original sinful nature.

Yes, my resume may be extensive, and yes I've held many titles---still do. But let me tell you, there's only one title I want God to acknowledge in that last day when I appear before Him. I want Him to say, "Well done my good and faithful servant."

It's very important to understand who we are in the sight of God, otherwise, we can't intersect with our purpose. Don't miss your godly purpose because of an identity crisis. Know who you are and who it is you belong to.

Don't be like that person on a merry-go-round, going around and around, or like a hamster running on the same wheel, day in and day out. Instead, acknowledge what the bible tells us in Psalm 37: 23-24: "The steps of a good man, (a good woman), are ordered by the Lord." I want God to order my steps, how about you?

Ironically, once you become a child of God, know who you are, whose you are, and where you're going, you'll discover that unfortunately, not everyone is happy for you. Other than in heaven or in church, you'll rarely find a clapping section for the children of God. After all, Lucifer himself was once a child of God. In fact, he was reportedly the chief musician, but because he thought he was better than God, he was kicked out of heaven by God Himself, and a third of the angels with him, never to return.

After you get saved, some people will be feeling some type of way towards you because they've lost their running buddy, their partner in crime, or their wing man. Your newfound joy and purpose makes them uncomfortable and resentful that you've left your old life behind. Mark my words however, they'll definitely see the change in you and over time will witness the power of God in you.

Eventually some will be won over by your testimony. Others will continue to serve the devil, but it's important to let our light shine before them so that they may see Christ in us.

We are not called to judge people or look down on anyone, we are simply called to lead the way towards salvation through Jesus Christ. The bible tells us to let our light shine before men so they may see Christ in us (and they will), and glorify God.

The Bible says to, "Choose you this day whom you will serve" (Joshua 24:14). There are times when we come face to face with that choice. Those still serving the devil can never have what we enjoy without first having Jesus. We've got Jesus, we've got the promise of heaven, we have abundant life. The sinful nature of the sinner is jealous and angry of what we have. Over time however, they will long for the peace, the joy, forgiveness, and the love they see in us.

SO WHY AM I HERE?

The Bible tells us in II Corinthians 5: 18-21, that we are ambassadors to Christ and that all of this is from God who reconciled us to himself through Jesus Christ and gave us the ministry of reconciliation.

WHAT IS MY PURPOSE?

When you know who you are, you begin to understand why you're here. God said He gave us a ministry of reconciliation, meaning He gave you a ministry of reconciliation. God reconciled the world to Himself in Christ, no longer counting men's trespasses against them. So, how can I count somebody's trespasses against them if God no longer holds my trespasses against me? How can I condemn someone else's trespasses if God has forgiven me of my own?

If you're wondering what's stopping your power, what's regulating your anointing? If you want to know why you're not walking in the power of reconciliation, it's most likely because you have unforgiveness in your heart. Stop judging everybody else and what they're doing wrong and focus instead on what you're doing or not doing. The Bible indicates that before you try taking a little pin out of my eye you need to remove the plank that's in your own (Matthew 7:5). The Bible does not tell us to work out Latonya's salvation, Marcel's salvation or Mom's salvation. Instead, it teaches us to work out our own salvation.

I go to the gym four days a week and to this day, I sometimes hate going because I know I'm the one who has to complete the workout. No one else can do it for me. Every time I plan on working out, I have to push myself to get there and when I get there, I have to force myself to complete my workout. But let me tell you, each time I finish working out, I feel great and I'm so glad I did it. So, you see, we can't work out anyone else's salvation, but we can lead the way to salvation through our example, remembering that judging others is of no use to us or them.

Your personal journey and resulting testimony become your purpose. God tells us that we go through hardships so that one day we may comfort someone else who is going through a similar hardship (2 Corinthians 1:4). Reassuring someone that you made it through and that they can too means so much, particularly when they're in the depths of pain or loss.

Every last one of us has a testimony. Every one of us has been through some fire. We've all been through some stuff. We've been knocked down, bruised, and messed up in some way. Jesus was blameless and without sin, yet He was bruised for our iniquities, but thanks be to God, by His stripes we are healed.

WHERE AM I GOING?

I'm not talking about a career choice, geographical location, or where I'm going to eat once I finish reading this section; I'm talking about eternity. The Bible teaches us that those of us who are going to heaven; those of us who have accepted Christ as our personal Lord and Savior, those of us who know who we are, and whose we are---know exactly where we're going.

For that reason, the first question we need to be asking ourselves is, "Am I going to heaven or am I going to hell?"

Because of God's great love for all mankind, He has given us a mandate. He said, "Go ye therefore and teach all nations baptizing them in the name of the Father and of the Son and of the Holy Ghost" (Matthew 8: 18-20). We've been given a mandate Saints of God so if you want to know your purpose, simply go and teach others what we've discovered. Our mandate in its simplest form is to tell others about Jesus by sharing the goodness of God and what He's done for you and for all mankind. It's to point the way to salvation and eternal life through Jesus Christ.

Psalms 34:19

"Many are the afflictions but the Lord delivered them from them all."

There is a reason for your pain. There is a reason why you used to run the streets. There's a reason you became an alcoholic. There's a reason why you were a liar or why someone hurt you or offended you. There's a reason why you went through a divorce. There's a reason why your children acted crazy out there in the streets and you couldn't seem to get them together. There was a reason for it all and the Bible tells us that, "many are our afflictions" (Psalm 34:19). Indeed! We've all been afflicted in some way. But you see, if we'd never been afflicted, we wouldn't know the power of God. There was a reason for your pain and there is a reason for your scars. What the devil meant for evil, God will use for good.

Your pain became your scars, Your scars became your healing and your healing became your purpose. Your purpose is your testimony, which is proof positive that God is able to deliver every one of us!

We who are called, "children of God," the sons and daughters of God, know that He's got all power in His hands. God has given us the answer for a world so wrought with; pain, homelessness, crime, anger, violence, and hatred. The bible teaches us that, "in the last days, men and women will be lovers of themselves," (11 Timothy 3: 1-5). They're going to love themselves more than they love God. We see it playing out right before our very eyes. People are self-centered and selfish and most only care about themselves.

We've been given the solution to reigning in wayward children, to fixing our bank accounts, the stock market, get jobs, buy houses, cars, etc. We have been given the blueprint to fix the city and the country. God said, "If I be lifted up, I'll draw all men unto me," (John 12: 32). "He is able to do exceedingly, abundantly above all that we can ever ask or think," (Ephesians 3: 20-21).

Our main purpose is to share the gospel and to spread the solution. And let me add, sharing the gospel is not simply preaching, quoting scripture or beating someone over the head with, "Thou ought to or ought not to!" Yes, we must be ready to share the path to salvation, but sharing the gospel is also about being kind, doing good deeds, giving someone a ride or meeting an urgent need.

Acts of kindness and service are a way to "Let our lives shine before men." Pray, "Lord, here I am, send me." And see where He leads you. He will put people in your path so you can let your light shine and share the gospel of Jesus Christ…He will create opportunities, so be ready to walk in your purpose and share the good news!

SCRIPTURE REFERENCES & RECAP

Mark 8:27-29

Peter Declares That Jesus Is the Messiah

"Jesus and His disciples went on to the villages around Caesarea Philippi. On the way He asked them, "Who do people say that I am?" They replied, "Some say John the Baptist; others say Elijah; and still others, one of the prophets. But what about you?" He asked. "Who do you say I am?" Peter answered, "You are the Messiah."

If we are Christians or call ourselves men and woman of God we have been made new.

2 Corinthians 5:17

"Therefore, if anyone is in Christ, the new creation has come: The old has gone, the new is here!"

The minute I accept Christ I am a new creation. However, if we're truly honest with ourselves, many of us still have the residue of our past hurt, pain, and scars that show up every day. Nevertheless, our experiences, which helped shape us into who we are today, have the possibility of becoming our testimonies.

We are ambassadors for Christ.

II Corinthians 5: 18-21

"All this is from God, who reconciled us to Himself through Christ and gave us the ministry of reconciliation: that God was reconciling the world to Himself in Christ, not counting men's trespasses against them. And He has committed to us the message of reconciliation.

Therefore, we are ambassadors for Christ, as though God were making His appeal through us. We implore you on behalf of Christ: Be reconciled to God. God made Him who knew no sin to be sin on our behalf, so that in Him we might become the righteousness of God."

Christ gave us a mandate:

Matthew 28:19

"Go ye therefore, and teach all nations, baptizing them in the name of the Father, and of the Son, and of the Holy Ghost."

Luke 14:23 (KJV)

"And the lord said unto the servant, go out into the highways and hedges, and compel them to come in, that my house may be filled."

NOTES

Do you know your God-Given purpose? Are you beginning to see God's plan for you?

_____
_____
_____
_____
_____
_____
_____
_____
_____
_____
_____
_____
_____
_____

PART 5

THE PRAISE

THE PRAISE

God dwells in the praises of His people. Praise lives inside us. We don't need a keyboard. We don't need a praise team because praise is in our hearts.

There are many reasons and many ways to praise God. There are so many things to thank Him for. Everything may not be perfect in our lives, but we can always find something to praise Him for. If nothing else, we can simply praise Him for who He is, for waking us up in the morning, and definitely for His unconditional love toward us.

Do you have joy in your heart today? Are you glad you know Jesus? Are you excited at the thought of how powerful He is? Happy about His mercy and Grace toward us?

The Lord is high above the heavens, and His glory shines above the nations. You are the healer, Lord. You're my provider. You are everything I need. You're my shelter, you're my keeper. You are a miracle worker, a way maker and a promise keeper. You give us strength when we have none. You give us love, when we feel unloved. You've never left us and in spite of any situation we've gone through God, you were right there.

We know you as a healer. We were broken, but you made us whole. We will exalt you and praise your name. You have done wonderful things for us. You are Lord, our strength and shield. Your loving kindness is better than life and my lips will glorify you. I will praise you as long as I live.

There are many examples in the bible where believers praised God despite their dire circumstances. It was about midnight when

Paul and Silas, while imprisoned, were praying and singing hymns to God despite the terrible situation they were in. The other prisoners heard them and were amazed and wondered how Paul and Silas could praise God at a time like that?

People are watching us too. They're watching to see how we're going to navigate our trials. Despite the fact that we endure the same sort of things they do, and live through similar situations, it's at those times when God's grace and power shine brightly through us. People soon realize there's something different about us. After all, thanks to the Holy Spirit, we are equipped to navigate our trials full of hope and praising God.

"I am fearfully and wonderfully made. Your works are wonderful. Great is the Lord and most worthy of praise. I will exalt the Lord at all times," (Psalm 139:14).

God can turn some of our most traumatic experiences into our greatest opportunities. It is often through pain, grief, and trials that God reveals His purpose for us; our purpose.

Trauma and pain are not the only way God reveals himself to us, but He will often manifest Himself through the pain. In fact, He declared "when we are weak, He is made strong." The fact that God is there during our greatest times of need, is simply more evidence of His great love for us. He is truly close to the broken-hearted.

As previously mentioned, the loss of my father was very traumatic for me, but in 1995 I received a distressing call indicating that my stepfather, an Orlando firefighter, had suddenly passed away. He'd drowned in a boating accident while fishing with his brothers in Tampa, Florida. They'd gone fishing and the boat capsized with him and his two brothers on board. His brothers survived the accident, but my stepfather had drowned.

A rescue helicopter was sent to retrieve his body and tragically, a police officer fell out of the helicopter and also drowned.

As a result, there were two first responder funerals in the same town, during the same week; one for a police officer and another for a firefighter, both having drowned in the same tragic accident.

My little brother who was my stepfather's only son was just 11 years old when my stepfather died. Not only was my mother distraught and grieving, but my little brother was too.

At that time, I was in the middle of a semester at Monroe Community College in Rochester, NY. It was definitely not at all good timing for me to stop attending school, particularly since

I'd just started using the G.I. Bill. I couldn't help but wonder "why had this happened to me now?"

I remember walking through the hallways completely distraught at the news I'd just received. Despite my educational journey, I knew my mother really needed me in Orlando.

While walking, I came across a poster on a wall indicating that Disney World was hiring. It promised that working at Disney meant I could continue to earn college credits while getting paid. I applied for the position and got the job. Wow, there I was receiving college credit, working for one of the best companies in the world, while thankfully able to care for my mother in her time of need.

A young man named Paul, who had traveled to Orlando with me from Rochester, took me to a Christian bookstore one day where I bought a tract (a comic book style pamphlet). It depicted a picture of heaven and a picture of hell. On the hell side, a huge crowd of people were falling off a cliff into a fiery pit while the road to heaven was depicted as a winding mountain road leading upward upon which few were traveling.

The pamphlet concluded by asking, "Which way do YOU want to go, heaven or hell?" I made a decision that day in the summer of 1995 right there in the Orlando Magic Mall parking lot, that I did not want to go to hell. I received Christ as my Lord and Savior which I formalized that following Sunday in the presence of my mother, in the church she attended.

Tragically and ironically, the gentleman who took me to the Christian bookstore and who ultimately led me to Christ, ended up backsliding later that summer. God showed me very early on that salvation is not so much about the people he uses, but ultimately about His great love for us. God can use anybody to lead us toward our destination and purpose. I've been serving God ever since.

SCRIPTURE REFERENCES & RECAP

The word *praise* appears in the King James Version of the bible 259 times.

Isaiah 25:1

"Let everything that has breath praise the Lord. Praise the Lord."

Psalm 150:6

"Praise the Lord, my soul;
all my inmost being, praise His holy name."

Psalm 103:1

"The Lord is my strength and my shield;
my heart trusts in Him, and He helps me.
My heart leaps for joy, and with my song I praise him."

Psalm 28:7

"I will give thanks to you, Lord, with all my heart; I will tell of all your wonderful deeds."

Psalm 9:1

"Because your love is better than life,
my lips will glorify you.
I will praise you as long as I live,
and in your name I will lift up my hands."

Psalm 63:3-4

"About midnight Paul and Silas were praying and singing hymns to God, and the other prisoners were listening to them."

Acts 16:25

"Why, my soul, are you downcast?
Why so disturbed within me?
Put your hope in God,

for I will yet praise Him,
my Savior and my God."

Psalm 42:11

"For you created my inmost being;
you knit me together in my mother's womb.
I praise you because I am fearfully and
wonderfully made;
your works are wonderful,
I know that full well."

Psalm 139:13-14

"Great is the Lord and most worthy of
praise; His greatness no one can fathom."

Psalm 145:3

"My mouth is filled with your praise,
declaring your splendor all day long."

Psalm 71:8

"Then I heard every creature in heaven and on earth and under the earth and on the sea, and all that is in them, saying: "To Him who sits on the throne and to the Lamb be praise and honor and glory and power, for ever and ever!"

Revelation 5:13

"I will extol the Lord at all times;
His praise will always be on my lips."

Psalm 34:1

"Let the message of Christ dwell among you richly as you teach and admonish one another with all wisdom through psalms, hymns, and songs from the Spirit, singing to God with gratitude in your hearts.

Colossians 3:16

"Give praise to the Lord, proclaim His name;
make known among the nations what He has done."

Psalm 105:1

"Finally, brothers and sisters, whatever is true, whatever is noble, whatever is right, whatever is pure, whatever is lovely, whatever is admirable—if anything is excellent or praiseworthy—think about such things."

Philippians 4:8

"It is written: 'As surely as I live,' says the Lord,
'every knee will bow before me;
every tongue will acknowledge God."

Romans 14:11

"I will exalt you, my God the King;
I will praise your name for ever and ever."
Psalm 145:1

"In that day you will say, give praise to the Lord, proclaim His name; make known among the nations what He has done,
and proclaim that His name is exalted."

Isaiah 12:4

"In God, whose word I praise—in God I trust and am not afraid. What can mere mortals do to me?"

Psalm 56:4

"Every day they continued to meet together in the temple courts. They broke bread in their homes and ate together with glad and sincere hearts, praising God and enjoying the favor of all the people. And the Lord added to their number daily those who were being saved."

Acts 2:46-47

"I will praise you with an upright heart
as I learn your righteous laws."

Psalm 119:7

"Heal me, Lord, and I will be healed;
save me and I will be saved,
for you are the one I praise."

Jeremiah 17:14

"I cried out to Him with my mouth;
His praise was on my tongue."

Psalm 66:17

I thank and praise you, God of my ancestors:
You have given me wisdom and power,

you have made known to me what we asked of you, you have made known to us the dream of the king."

Daniel 2:23

"I will praise you, Lord, among the nations;
I will sing of you among the peoples."

Psalm 119:105

"Your word is a lamp for my feet, a light on my path."

Regardless of where you may be along this journey towards the intersection between pain and purpose, it's important to rely on what the scriptures tell us.

In Romans 12:2, we are told: "Do not conform to the pattern of this world, but be ye transformed by the renewing of your mind.

Then you will be able to test and approve what God's will is, His good, pleasing and perfect will."

Romans 8:28 teaches, "And we know that all things work together for good to them that love God and who are called according to His purpose."

It's important that we understand that it's the renewing of the mind that leads us to that place of purpose. Note that even though we are a new creation in Christ, the "renewing of the mind" is an ongoing process. Along this journey and process, we must understand that our thoughts have the capacity to be renewed every day.

The Bible indicates that regardless of where we are in our journey we must rest assured that the steadfast love of the Lord never ceases and there is no end to His mercy. In fact, His mercies are new every morning and great is His faithfulness.

Starting today, make it a good day and understand that you will arrive at the intersection of your pain and your purpose because, "All things work together for the good for them who are called according to His purpose." Remember that our purpose as children of God is ultimately to align with God's purpose for us.

NOTES

What does praise look like for you?

WILLIE J. LIGHTFOOT SR.

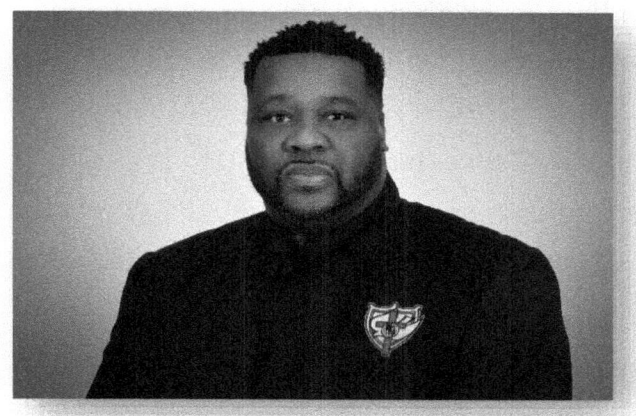

ABOUT THE AUTHOR

From a young age, Willie J. Lightfoot Sr. has been invested in our community. As the son of Theresa Thompson and The Late Honorable Willie Walker Lightfoot, 25th District County Legislator for more than 20 years, Willie J. Lightfoot Sr. is no stranger to politics and the concept of community service.

It's no surprise that Willie J. Lightfoot Sr. was appointed to the Monroe County Legislature in 2006. He represented Monroe County's 27th District which encompasses the Frederick Douglas Greater Rochester International Airport, Rochester's diverse 19th Ward neighborhood, and Genesee Valley Park. He termed out after three consecutive terms, serving a total of 10 years as a County Legislator.

Lightfoot is currently a City Councilman at large. He was the ranking Democrat on the Public Safety Committee and also served on the Human Services Committee. Mr. Lightfoot, along with his wife Verdina, have four adult children and three grandchildren. A lifelong resident of the City of Rochester, LIghtfoot often refers to himself as "Home Grown."

Willie J. Lightfoot Sr. has a long history of civic service. He is a 12-year Veteran of the United States Air Force. He served in two wars;

Desert Storm and Operation Enduring Freedom. Lightfoot is also a retired City of Rochester firefighter. He is a 2005 graduate of the African American Leadership Development Program (AALDP), and a 2007 graduate of Leadership Rochester.

Willie J. Lightfoot Sr. sat on the following boards: Center for Dispute Settlement, Jefferson Avenue Childhood Development, and His Branches, a neighborhood medical family practice.
Lightfoot was appointed to the Monroe County Airport Authority Board and the Monroe County Fire Advisory Board. Willie is the founder of the *Cut The Violence Initiative,* which helps curb teen violence in the Rochester area. He has received numerous community awards and recognitions.

Willie J. Lightfoot Sr. and Verdina are proud members of the 19th Ward Community Association. Willie is the owner of a Real Estate Investment company called OHAD, which is a Hebrew name which means, *loved one*.

He is the developer of *LIGHTFOOT SQUARE* a 4,500 square foot multi-purpose building. Willie is a NYS licensed Barber and a NYS Barber Examiner/ Supervisor. He owns and operates his own Unisex shop, *New Creations Unisex*.

It's not uncommon for customers and barbers alike to engage at the barbershop in meaningful discussions surrounding the needs and the future of our community. That's how Lightfoot likes it, as it allows him to hear from and keep a pulse on the community he serves. Mr. Lightfoot is an ordained Elder and is the Pastor of *Prayer House Church of God By Faith*. He earned two Associates degrees; one from Monroe Community College in Business Administration and the other from the Community College of the Air Force for Fire Science. He also holds a Bachelor's Degree from Empire State College.

If that's not enough, he is the Founder and President of United Professional Barbers and Cosmetologists Association (UPBCA). This association was created to support small businesses and provide benefits to barbers and cosmetologists throughout Monroe County.

Willie J. Lightfoot Sr. enjoys reading, listening to music and traveling. He loves his community and the people therein and is a proud Rochesterian. He is often referred to as *Rochester's Son* because everybody knows and respects him.

NATIONAL MENTAL HEALTH RESOURCES & SUPPORT ORGANIZATIONS

https://www.fcc.gov/988-suicide-and-crisis-lifeline

Today, **"988"** is the three-digit, nationwide phone number to connect directly to the **988 Suicide and Crisis Lifeline.** By calling or texting 988, you'll connect with mental health professionals with the 988 Suicide and Crisis Lifeline, formerly known as the National Suicide Prevention Lifeline. Veterans can press "1" after dialing 988 to connect directly to the Veterans Crisis Lifeline which serves our nation's Veterans, service members, National per (www.fcc.com).

https://www.nimh.nih.gov/health/find-help

The National Institute of Mental Health (NIMH), website has lots of helpful information, resources and can help you find a trained professional in your area.

www.namica.org

The National Alliance on Mental Illness (NAMI) is a national mental health organization/hotline. There are offices in every state and in most cities. They have support groups, offer advice and a list of local resources to meet your specific needs.

www.ingramcontent.com/pod-product-compliance
Lightning Source LLC
Chambersburg PA
CBHW071313110426
42743CB00042B/1623